Food

Is It Really about Our Health?

*Finding Hope with
Cancer and Disease*

ALAN FORTIN

ISBN 979-8-89309-055-0 (Paperback)
ISBN 979-8-89309-056-7 (Digital)

Copyright © 2024 Alan Fortin
All rights reserved
First Edition

All rights reserved. No part of this publication may be reproduced, distributed, or transmitted in any form or by any means, including photocopying, recording, or other electronic or mechanical methods without the prior written permission of the publisher. For permission requests, solicit the publisher via the address below.

Covenant Books
11661 Hwy 707
Murrells Inlet, SC 29576
www.covenantbooks.com

CONTENTS

Preface v
Introduction vii

Chapter 1: Why So Many Cancers? 1
Chapter 2: What Is a Healthy Diet? 3
Chapter 3: Immune System 6
Chapter 4: Pesticides in Agriculture 9
Chapter 5: Genetically Modified Organisms (GMOs)
 in Agriculture 16
Chapter 6: Hormones in Agriculture 19
Chapter 7: Organic versus Nonorganic 21
Chapter 8: Food Labels 22
Chapter 9: World Health Organization (WHO) 25
Chapter 10: Sugars 26
Chapter 11: Foods in the Bible 31
Chapter 12: My Cup of Tea 33
Chapter 13: Herbs and Spices 35
Chapter 14: Omega-3 Fatty Acids 42
Chapter 15: Beef: Grass-Fed versus Grain-Fed 44
Chapter 16: Fruits and Nuts 45

Conclusion 47

PREFACE

SINCE I HAVE impaired vision from the radiation treatment, I can no longer drive, so work is extremely limited. However, I still want to provide for my family, so I thought I'd write this book to not only help my family but perhaps help yours too.

Looking back at my childhood, I believed all foods were good for you, or at least wouldn't hurt you. I thought, why would they sell unhealthy food, and why would we buy them? Especially if they could make us sick or worse. As I became older, I realized it's not entirely about the consumers' health but profits in the food industry and investors on Wall Street too.

I became convinced that it was my responsibility to eat the proper food, and so my journey began. It wasn't until my grandchildren asked, "Poppy, how do you know what foods are good for you?"

Then it dawned on me, and I answered, "If God made it, then it's good for you. If man made it, it's probably not." That discussion led to a quiz. I asked the children if an apple was healthy.

They all thought and answered proudly, "Yes, Poppy, an apple is good for you, because God made it."

I then asked if oranges, bananas, and vegetables were healthy.

They were all proud to answer, saying, "Since God made them, then they're good for you."

It wasn't until I asked about the Cheetos they were eating that they became concerned. They answered with a hopeful glee, "Good for you!" Did you know Cheetos are identified as an unhealthy snack? I didn't either.

However, after learning about hormones, genetically modified organisms (GMOs), as well as pesticides, herbicides, and other chemicals used on our food and in our soil, I am no longer sure that God's food is still healthy since they've either been modified or treated with chemicals, and in some cases, both.

I came to this realization after reading about hormones, as well as genetically modified organisms (GMOs) and pesticides entering the food system. I became sad, disturbed, and disappointed with the FDA, EPA, and to some degree, the financial market on Wall Street since I believe allowing chemicals and modifying food was driven by financial gain and not our health.

I do not want to scare anyone from eating, but I feel it's best to be informed so we, the families, can be comfortable and confident with the foods we buy and eat. Like the saying goes, we are what we eat, and our health reflects that.

INTRODUCTION

I HAVE BEEN dealing with stage 4 glioblastoma since August 30, 2021. So attempting to write my first book has been quite challenging, but I find it therapeutic. And besides, I always liked a challenge. My vision has been damaged from the radiation treatment, and I lost sight left of center in both eyes, so typing, which has never been very good, makes it at times frustrating as well as discouraging. But I've realized I am either stubborn, determined, or perhaps both, because I always seem to continue. As you read this book, you'll probably see how my mind drifts due to the disease, but hopefully, after many proofreads, you can find it to be informative and enjoyable. Writing this book required a lot of research, and through that research, I learned so many things that I used to take for granted.

A brief snapshot of my health throughout my life may help provide a better understanding of why I wrote this book.

- At six years of age, I became totally blind for a few hours. Then presto, my vision returned, although very poor.
- In 1975, at seventeen years old, I was diagnosed with Dupuytren's contracture disease, better known as Viking's disease.
- In March 1995, I was diagnosed with Clark's level 4 melanoma.
- June 2018: basal cell carcinoma.
- August 30, 2021: stage 4 glioblastoma brain cancer.

What a day to be diagnosed, on my mother's birthday.

Yikes! I thought. Another cancer! How many different cancers am I going to have? What did I do wrong? Could I have done something different? After my research, I realized and believe I could have, but it's impossible to know for sure if it would've made a difference. As you read this book, you'll see we all have many of the same challenges, but how you handle it, hopefully, has a better outcome than the way I did.

CHAPTER 1

Why So Many Cancers?

As I mentioned in the introduction, I've had my share of various cancers. But why so many, and why are they all different? None had metastasized, just a different cancer diagnosed each time.

Malignant melanoma

The exact cause of melanoma isn't clear, but it is believed to be the result of too much exposure to UV rays, like those in tanning beds and the sun.

Basal cell carcinoma

This skin cancer is also believed to be caused by too much UV radiation and sun exposure.

Glioblastoma

The cause of glioblastoma is still unknown. However, researchers have found a link with burn pits, to which I have been exposed while overseas. Also, a cure has not yet been identified, but I still have hope. The reason for my hope is that I believe my immune system is improving, and besides, without hope, there's no desire. I have plenty of both and want to share with you in this book how you can have both too.

As a child and throughout most of my life, being outside was my favorite place to be, so I can see where sun exposure could play a part in two of my cancers. I was either swimming with family or friends, bailing hay, or straw for extra money in the summer, playing ball, and in high school, running 120 miles a week to feed my competitiveness in track and cross country. My goals were to break the 4-minute mile and win gold at the Olympics. Unfortunately, my feet aren't designed for running; I always walk on the outside of my feet, so the long distances of running eventually fractured a bone in my foot from the constant torque. After recovering from the fracture, I was still able to run a 4:16 mile on a loose cinder track, but I knew I wasn't in the shape I could have been in if the fracture had never occurred. Close, but no cigar. The world record at the time was 3:51.

After school, I joined the military and performed aircraft inspections using UV lights and aircraft parts using high-powered electromagnetic fields, a process called magnetic particle inspection. Perhaps that had something to do with glioblastoma as well as skin cancers? I don't know.

I mentioned my exposures because I still believe I could have improved my chances of not getting cancer or Dupuytren's contracture disease by eating a healthier diet and improving my immune system.

CHAPTER 2

What Is a Healthy Diet?

I DIDN'T THINK about nutritional value until later in life. I thought a nice balanced diet was the best way to go, but what does that mean? Don't have too much of any one thing? What about fruit and vegetables or meat and fish? So I'd eat some kind of meat, instant potatoes, and some kind of vegetable then snack on anything I wanted, as long as it wasn't too much. I even researched healthy foods to eat, and a list of different diets came up, such as balanced diet, Mediterranean diet, keto diet, plant-based diet, gluten-free diet, low-fat diet, etc. Just so many to choose from. But to me, diet meant you wanted to lose weight, and I didn't want to lose weight. I just wanted to eat good, nutritional foods. However, the more research I did, the more concerned I became, because I didn't realize how much the foods we eat have been treated with chemicals and hormones and modified using genetically modified organisms (GMOs). To me, eating healthfully became confusing and rather difficult to know for sure if I was eating foods to help or hurt me. I'll explain why in the upcoming chapters. Please keep in mind I'm writing this book with stage 4 glioblastoma, and my mind gets a bit confused as I try putting my thoughts on paper. Multitasking has become very difficult with this disease.

My wife, who has been fantastic in this battle of fighting cancer with me, does everything. The radiation damage to my vision prevents me from driving, so she does all the driving, shopping, and cooking. She's perfect and always a comforter. Her steadfast love and support are so encouraging, which inspires me to keep moving on. When I was first diagnosed with glioblastoma, she recommended a naturopathic doctor who I used once before. He provides so much guidance on which foods I should eat and foods to avoid based on the genetic makeup of my body. He also suggested certain supplements and juicing, which is also based on my genetic makeup and needs. So my diet now consists of a lot of omega-3 fatty acids, which I get by eating grass-fed beef, lamb, and venison as well as wild-caught salmon and some other fish too. The Bible mentions fish with scales and fins, so I'm okay with any fish that fit in that category as well. I also eat a lot of oranges and red grapes to satisfy my sweet tooth, but sadly I found those fruits were identified in the Dirty Dozen (https://foodrevolution.org). This website has wonderful information to help us make more informed decisions on what food choices we can make in our attempt to eat healthier by listing what produce has the most and least amount of toxins detected.

In addition, I love dark chocolate; however, recent news mentioned arsenic was in some dark chocolate. I'd eat dark chocolate with a handful of nuts (almonds, Brazil nuts, pecans, and sunflower seeds) as a snack. Instead of calling it a balanced diet, keto, low-fat, plant-based, or gluten-free diet, I think I'll just call it Alan's diet. After all, the average survival for stage 4 glioblastoma is 12 to 18 months from diagnosis and only 5 percent of patients survive more than 5 years. Also, the average time for a recurrence is 9.5 months from diagnosis, and I'm alive with no recurrence at 27 months. I have been blessed with a wonderful team of doctors who have made the right call every time. Having *hope* is so critical when battling such a deadly disease, and I believe I have found my hope through God, doctors, family, diet, and friends.

Could I have prevented all these cancers? Perhaps. If I had eaten the right foods to strengthen my immune system, I believe it could have helped to fight off my disease and cancers better than not having a good immune system. Proving that is probably impossible, but it does make sense, which is why I believe it is possible. Is it now too late? No! I'm still alive, feeling well, and following a diet plan recommended by my naturopath to strengthen and maintain a healthy

FOOD

immune system. I know I can't live forever on earth, but even with cancers and disease, I want the remainder of my life to be as healthy as I can make it. It's my choice, and I'm up for the challenge.

CHAPTER 3

Immune System

WHAT IS THE immune system anyway? It's your body's natural ability to fight off sickness and disease. When your immune system is weak, it allows bad cells to continue to get worse. I believe when symptoms occur, most people seek medical attention and are usually prescribed medications. However, in my case, surgery was prescribed to remove three different tumors in my lifetime. Keep in mind, medications and operations do nothing to improve your immune system. Could I have done something different to help my body fight off cancer, disease, viruses, and sickness? I believe I could have done better. I believe we all can.

Can the immune system be hereditary? Yes, a study conducted at Kings College, London, revealed that nearly three-quarters of immune traits are influenced by genes. As an example, my mother unfortunately passed from Parkinson's disease, her mom passed from atherosclerosis disease, and her grandmother passed from tuberculosis. Could I have the genes from my mother's side? I don't know, but of four brothers, I am the only child affected by diseases. I still believe, however, that I could have improved my chances of fighting diseases and cancers by improving my immune system.

I've never been a doctor, and I am not going to pretend I am now. I am simply looking at my own experiences and writing what I believe could have made a difference.

How is your immune system? Your doctor or a naturopath should be able to let you know the status of your immune system and provide guidance or additional information.

Can we improve our immune system? Yes (https://www.indushealthplus.com/genetic-dna-testing/genetics-reason-behind-good-immune-system.html). As your immune system is influenced by your DNA, the blueprint of your life, you can strive to make changes in your lifestyle (including food and exercise) to achieve a healthier life and stronger immune response. By understanding your genetic tendencies, you can take appropriate corrective actions to improve and strengthen your immune system and its functions. Although genetic tests are available for purchase online, I suggest having a conversation with your doctor first. I believe doctors will be happy to see you being proactive in your health and will gladly support you.

A recent article from the University of Penn Medicine discusses the immune system and how it can prevent every type of disease (https://www.pennmedicine.org/news/publications-and-special-projects/penn-medicine-magazine/immune-health/the-immune-health-future-today). Breaking the code of the immune system could provide a new fundamental way of understanding, treating, and preventing every type of disease. Penn Medicine is investing in key discoveries about immunity and immune system function and building infrastructure to make that bold idea a reality.

Why not do our part too by eating the right food? But what are the right foods, and are they safe to eat? Unfortunately, after reading what might be in our food supply, how do you know the vegetables, fruit, and meat we're eating aren't loaded with pesticides, GMOs, chemicals, or hormones? The next chapter will mention my concerns in further detail, and the chapter on labels will help you shop with confidence.

It's sad to even talk about this, but after reviewing so much info, it just seems more likely than not that our food isn't as good for us as I once thought.

I just received a text from a friend whose wife was just diagnosed with cancer. Of the treatments she needs, one of her first is a booster shot for her immune system. That text made me think maybe this is just another reason why I should write this book, so perhaps we can stay in front of disease and cancer instead of reacting.

Science, in the medical field, has numerous clinical trials using immunotherapy to treat diseases and cancers, so why not get in front of diseases and cancers and improve our own immune system? I wish I did. But to improve our immune system, we also need to know about the foods considered to be healthy. To lead into the next chapter, I'll ask a simple question. Are you concerned about toxins, hormones, or GMOs in our food supply? I am, and the next chapter will explain why.

If I weren't concerned about toxins, hormones, or GMOs, then I would probably just follow the advice to shop only on the outside aisles at the grocery store. But I do have concerns, and the next chapter will show why.

CHAPTER 4

Pesticides in Agriculture

WHAT ARE PESTICIDES, and why are they applied to vegetation?

A pesticide is any substance or mixture of substances intended for preventing, destroying, repelling, or mitigating any pest. Pesticides are used in agriculture to protect crops from insects, fungi, weeds, and other pests. Federal government agencies in the United States share responsibility for the oversight of pesticide chemical residues in or on food. The Environmental Protection Agency (EPA) evaluates pesticides to ensure that they are safe for human health and the environment when used according to label directions.

Do health concerns exist with the consumption of pesticide application to vegetation? Yes, according to (https://www.ehn.org/pesticides-2659319421.html). Numerous studies have shown that consuming foods high in pesticide residue can increase the risk of certain health problems. Also, residues of some pesticides are more toxic than others. Numerous studies have been done on pesticides and their relation to cancers, but the results aren't conclusive. However, after more research, it looks like pesticides can play a role in skin cancers as well as cancers affecting the nervous system, including the brain. Hmmm, the three cancers I've been diagnosed with now have one common link: pesticides. But why? I only baled hay on a farm, and that was only occasionally. Could it be in the food I ate or eat? I don't know but thought it was worth exploring and sharing with you. After all, the grocery store wouldn't sell anything that is unhealthy, right? Even the government is making sure everything is safe to eat. Why should I worry? Maybe it's more about profit than it is about our health.

What do the following pesticides have in common? The suffix *-cide* means "killing" or "killer." That's the definition given on www.rxlist.com.

- Pesticide: Pesticides are any substance or mixture of substances intended for preventing, destroying, repelling, or mitigating any pest.
- Herbicide (https://www.epa.gov/caddis-vol2/herbicides): Herbicides are chemicals used to manipulate or control undesirable vegetation. Herbicide application occurs most frequently in row-crop farming where they are applied before or during planting to maximize crop productivity by minimizing other vegetation. They also may be applied to crops in the fall, to improve harvesting.
- Insecticide (https://www.epa.gov/caddis-vol2/insecticides): Insecticides are chemicals used to control insects by killing them or preventing them from engaging in undesirable or destructive behaviors. They are classified based on their structure and mode of action. Many insecticides act upon the insect's nervous system (e.g., cholinesterase inhibition) while others act as growth regulators or endotoxins.
- Fungicide (https://www.britannica.com/science/fungicide): Any toxic substance used to kill or inhibit the growth of fungi. Fungicides are generally used to control parasitic fungi that either cause economic damage to crop or ornamental plants or endanger the health of domestic levels animals or humans. Most agricultural and horticultural fungicides are applied as sprays or dusts.
- Rodenticide (http://npic.orst.edu/factsheets/rodenticides.html): Rodenticides are pesticides that kill rodents and include not only rats and mice but also squirrels, woodchucks, chipmunks, porcupines, nutria, and beavers. Although rodents play important roles in nature, they

may sometimes require control. They can damage crops, violate housing codes, transmit disease, and in some cases cause ecological damage. Rodents, humans, dogs, and cats are all mammals, so our bodies work in very similar ways. Rodenticides have the same effect when eaten by any mammal. They can also affect birds.

Since the use of chemicals has contaminated some soils, my fear is that vegetables and/or fruit can still be grown in contaminated soil. Pesticides have also found their way into bodies of water from runoff. Another fear now becomes, what toxins are in the fish we eat?

Are samples of food taken to recall food items due to elevated toxin levels, or are they just placed on the grocery store shelf?

Here's something I never tried but thought I'd share because I think it's a lot healthier than store-bought insect repellent. If rosemary, basil, and lavender do not cause allergies, then perhaps boiling one of them in water and using it as a spray will work just as well as insect repellent since insects don't like the scent. I'm sure it'll be less toxic than the pesticide repellent currently being sold.

Since the long-term health effects of consuming vegetation treated with pesticides are still unknown, I will make my own judgment. Consuming vegetation treated with pesticides is probably not healthy, and I believe the consumers should be informed by seeing a warning label on the package to let them know about the possible risks. Imagine the shock to see a warning label on a package of strawberries stating strawberries have been found to have the highest levels of toxins. Maybe a label should read, "Eat at your own risk." Either way, the consumer should know what their family is eating. Reference: (https://sitn.hms.harvard.edu/flash/2015/gmos-and-pesticides).

Pesticides have been used in farming for a long time. Early on, farmers used what was naturally available like pine straw, food waste, and other organic plants, fish bones, and even animal horns, which includes sulfur and, *yikes*, arsenic. Synthetic pesticides were first applied to vegetation in the 1930s. Genetically modified organisms (GMOs) were introduced in the 1990s to include pesticide agents.

Summary

Pesticides are ubiquitous. Because they are used in agriculture and food production, pesticides are present at low levels in many of our diets. Less obvious is the fact that many people use pesticides around their homes, and even on their skin using insect repellents. Not well understood, potential effects include cancer and damage to the nervous, endocrine, and reproductive systems.

Since the long-term effects of hormones, GMOs, and pesticides seem to be unknown, I did more research, and the more I explored, the more it concerned me. Pesticides seem to be everywhere: crops, lawns, water, and air when used as crop dusting or aerosol, such as insect repellent and who knows what else. The EPA has also identified some areas to be considered toxic waste cleanup sites. As a child, I recall a peach tree farmer about four miles down the road from where I lived at the time who sold his land to a developer to build homes. However, before they could build, they had to remove several feet of soil because the EPA said the soil was too toxic. What's sad is that we and others bought peaches there. How were we to know the peach trees were growing in toxic soil? I later learned from my sister-in-law that the farmer was her grandfather, and his son, her uncle, died from brain cancer. Another sister-in-law, who lived nearby, recalled seeing large sprayers in the orchard. No one knew what they were spraying. Other farmland in my area was known to have arsenic in its soil. What can we possibly do to help us in our attempt at healthy eating? What can we do to minimize our risk?

To reduce our exposure to pesticides and other chemicals, it is recommended to do the following:

- Buy organic produce.
- Thoroughly wash all fruit and vegetables (even organic).
- Grow your own vegetables.
- Peel leafy vegetables or remove the outer layer of leaves.

Know what's been tested and buy the food identified with the least amount of toxins (www.ewg.org). The Dirty Dozen lists produce with the highest levels of toxins, while the clean fifteen shows the lowest amount of toxins. Is consumption of fruit and vegetables, organic or not, critical to a healthy diet and good health? This is sad, especially when toddlers are encouraged to eat the following.

The 2023 Dirty Dozen

Of the forty-six items included in our analysis, these twelve fruits and vegetables were most contaminated:

1. Strawberries
2. Spinach
3. Kale, collard, and mustard greens
4. Peaches
5. Pears
6. Nectarines
7. Apples
8. Grapes
9. Bell and hot peppers
10. Cherries
11. Blueberries
12. Green beans

Some highlights from the Dirty Dozen testing:

- More than 90 percent of samples of strawberries, apples, cherries, spinach, nectarines, and grapes tested positive for residues of two or more pesticides.
- A total of 210 pesticides were found on Dirty Dozen items.
- Of those, over 50 different pesticides were detected on every type of crop on the list, except cherries.
- All the produce on the Dirty Dozen had at least one sample with at least 13 different pesticides—and some had as many as 23.

- Kale, collard, and mustard greens, as well as hot peppers and bell peppers, had the most pesticides detected of any crop—103 and 101 pesticides in total, respectively.
- The neurotoxic organophosphate insecticide acephate, prohibited from use on green beans in 2011, was detected in 6 percent of green bean samples.

If you're disheartened by the foods listed in the Dirty Dozen, please know you're not alone.

Here we are, my wife and I, doing everything we can to eat healthy not only to improve my immune system but also to try and beat an incurable stage 4 glioblastoma brain cancer. Instead, I'm eating all the foods that are most contaminated with pesticides. How is this even possible? Is food only about profit? Does our health even matter? Seems something in the food and health industry is broken if grocery stores are able to sell toxic foods for us to eat.

Perhaps since the food industry is a significant sector in the US economy with an estimated worth of over $1.5 trillion, maybe it's all about Wall Street making profit instead? But what do I know, I'm just someone trying to eat healthy. Perhaps it's the healthy foods that gave me cancer? I'd love someone to prove the toxins in and on the foods aren't the reason why I or anyone else has glioblastoma. Thank God the Environmental Working Group (EWG), a nonprofit group, is making us aware. Otherwise, I'd keep eating toxic food believing it's healthy.

So, since the '60s when I would go grocery shopping with Mom and thought everything in the store was healthy, it appears nothing has changed. That is incredibly sad, and I can't imagine why it's been ignored except by a group who are funded by donations, the EWG.

The 2023 Clean Fifteen

These fifteen items had the lowest amounts of pesticide residues, according to EWG's analysis of the most recent USDA data (https://www.ewg.org/foodnews):

1. Avocados
2. Sweet corn
3. Pineapple
4. Onions
5. Papaya
6. Sweet peas (frozen)
7. Asparagus
8. Honeydew melon
9. Kiwi
10. Cabbage
11. Mushrooms
12. Mangoes
13. Sweet potatoes
14. Watermelon
15. Carrots

Top takeaways for consumers:

- Almost 65 percent of Clean Fifteen fruit and vegetable samples had no detectable pesticide residues.
- Avocados and sweet corn were the cleanest produce—less than 2 percent of samples showed any detectable pesticides.
- Just over 10 percent of Clean Fifteen fruit and vegetable samples had residues of two or more pesticides.
- No sample from the first six Clean Fifteen items tested positive for more than three pesticides.

It breaks my heart to see some of the foods I'm eating right now on the high toxin list identified in the Dirty Dozen, especially when we've been thinking we were doing great fighting glioblastoma cancer by eating healthy foods.

Perhaps some people know the risks already, but there are so many unknowns with pesticides, I don't see how anyone could know them all. I noticed that thicker skin on vegetables and fruit held up better not to absorb chemicals than thin-skinned. Hopefully, by the time I finish this book, we'll have a more confident food plan.

CHAPTER 5

Genetically Modified Organisms (GMOs) in Agriculture

(https://www.fda.gov/food/agricultural-biotechnology/
science-and-history-gmos-and-other-food-modification-processes)

1922: THE FIRST hybrid corn is produced and sold commercially.
1940: Plant breeders learn to use radiation or chemicals to randomly change an organism's DNA.
1953: Building on the discoveries of chemist Rosalind Franklin, scientists James Watson and Francis Crick identify the structure of DNA.
1973: Biochemists Herbert Boyer and Stanley Cohen develop genetic engineering by inserting DNA from one bacteria into another.
1982: FDA approves the first consumer GMO product developed through genetic engineering: human insulin to treat diabetes.
1986: The federal government establishes the Coordinated Framework for the Regulation of Biotechnology. This policy describes how the US Food and Drug Administration (FDA), US Environmental Protection Agency (EPA), and US Department of Agriculture (USDA) work together to regulate the safety of GMOs.

What's concerning about this timeline is that the regulation of GMO safety didn't start until the 1980s, even though it was widely used since the 1940s.

The biggest threat caused by GMO foods is that they can have harmful effects on the human body. It is believed that the consumption of these genetically engineered foods can cause the development of diseases that are immune to antibiotics. Besides, since these foods are relatively new inventions, not much is known about their long-term health effects. As the health effects are unknown, many people prefer to stay away from these foods. Manufacturers/producers do not mention that foods are developed by genetic manipulation because they think that this would affect their business.

New studies are being done to determine how to use GMOs in animals too. I think that is beyond scary.

Scientists are developing new ways to create new varieties of crops and animals using a process called genome editing. These techniques can make changes more quickly and precisely than traditional breeding methods. There are several genome editing tools, such as CRISPR. Scientists can use these newer genome editing tools to make crops more nutritious, drought-tolerant, and resistant to insect pests and diseases.

Do you trust GMOs are safe in vegetation or animals?

Reference: (https://www.fda.gov/food/agricultural-biotechnology/why-do-farmers-us-grow-gmo-crops).

Most of the GMO crops grown today were developed to help farmers prevent crop and food loss and control weeds.

The three most common traits found in GMO crops are the following:

1. Resistance to certain damaging insects
2. Tolerance of certain herbicides is used to control weeds
3. Resistance to certain plant viruses

As an update to my condition of battling glioblastoma brain cancer, my vision seems to be getting worse. It seems my short-term memory is drifting away, and I continue to be tired most of the time. However, the stubbornness in me to continue is still active.

I know chapters 4, 5, and 6 are painful to read, but I want the best for you and your family so you can live a healthier life. These chapters are written to inform you of what's going on with the food we eat because, honestly, I never knew.

CHAPTER 6

Hormones in Agriculture

As if pesticides and GMOs didn't alarm me, I sadly discovered hormones and their health risks (https://www.ncbi.nlm.nih.gov/pmc/articles/PMC4524299).

The collected data from other researchers and our own data indicate that the presence of steroid hormones in dairy products could be counted as an important risk factor for various cancers in humans.

Why are hormones found in food?

Hormones are used for several reasons in animal-based food production, such as the following:

- Young animals gain weight faster
- Reduced waiting time
- Reduction in the average amount of feed required by an animal
- Increased milk production
- Increased overall efficiency and profitability of meat and dairy industries

In the US, there are six different kinds of hormones approved by the Food and Drug Administration (FDA) for use in food production. These include the naturally occurring female sex hormones estradiol and progesterone, natural male sex hormone testosterone, and three man-made chemicals zeranol, trenbolone acetate, and melengesterol acetate.

It is currently believed that the majority of hormones found in milk are transferred by diffusion. The most important hormones found in milk and other dairy products include the following:

- Prolactin
- Estrogen
- Progesterone
- Corticoids
- Androgens

CHAPTER 7

Organic versus Nonorganic

Organic

THE TERM *ORGANIC* refers to the way agricultural products are grown and processed. While the regulations vary from country to country, in the US, organic crops must be grown without the use of synthetic herbicides, pesticides, fertilizers, or bioengineered genes (GMOs).

Organic livestock raised for meat, eggs, and dairy products must be raised in living conditions accommodating their natural behaviors (such as the ability to graze on pasture) and fed organic feed and forage. They may not be given antibiotics, growth hormones, or any animal by-products.

Nonorganic

Nearly 75 percent of nonorganic fresh produce sold in the US contains residues of potentially harmful pesticides, with blueberries and green beans being added to the group's 2023 Dirty Dozen list, which names the top 12 fruits and vegetables with the most pesticide traces found.

The nonprofit health organization said on the website that the purpose of releasing an updated annual shopper's guide is to help consumers make safer, more informed food selections when buying produce for themselves or their families.

CHAPTER 8

Food Labels

THIS CHAPTER SHOULD help you to understand what to look for when trying to buy the healthiest foods for your family (https://foodprint.org/eating-sustainably/food-label-guide/).

Not all labels are created equal.

Some are clear indications that the food has been certified to meet certain requirements, such as "USDA Organic Certification" or "Animal Welfare Approved." Some, like "Pasture Raised," suggest certain standards were met or practices were used, but do not guarantee it. Sometimes the words themselves—as in the case of the word *natural*—have ceased to have any true meaning. That's why a comprehensive food label guide can be so useful.

Maybe these labels can be your guide in the supermarket aisle and at the farmers' market, leading you to food that has been raised and produced in a way that aligns with your values.

FOOD

Common labels

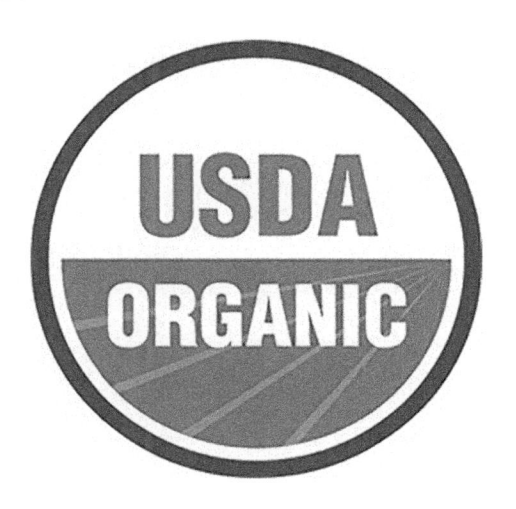

USDA Organic is a top pick

The organic label has among the strongest standards for environmental sustainability including prohibiting synthetic fertilizers and industrial pesticides. Animal feed must be 100 percent organically produced and without animal by-products or daily drugs. GMOs are prohibited (though testing is not required).

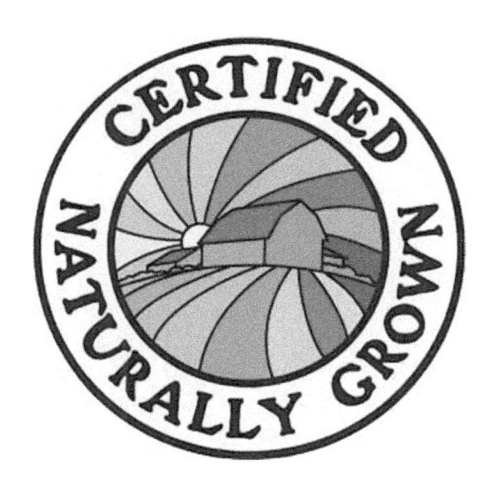

This label was started by farmers who did not want to go through USDA organic certification requirements. The label generally follows the USDA organic standards, but the verification is done by CNG farmers instead of independent certifiers.

CHAPTER 9

World Health Organization (WHO)

Reference: (https://www.who.int/news/item/02-07-2001-fao-who-call-for-more-international-collaboration-to-solve-food-safety-and-quality-problems).

GOVERNMENTS ACROSS THE globe urgently need to upgrade their domestic food safety systems, WHO and FAO (Food and Agriculture Organization) said. In many developing countries, there is often no comprehensive food safety system in place at all.

Since foods are provided globally from various countries, do the foods we eat from other countries follow the same standards and testing?

Some of the older, less costly pesticides can remain in soil and water for years. Many of these chemicals have been banned from agricultural use in developed countries, but they are still used in many developing countries.

Pesticides play a significant role in food production. They protect or increase yields and may increase the number of times each year a crop can be grown on the same land. This is particularly important in countries that face food shortages.

CHAPTER 10

Sugars

Reference: (https://www.health.harvard.edu/heart-health/the-sweet-danger-of-sugar).

SUGAR HAS A bittersweet reputation when it comes to health. Sugar occurs naturally in all foods that contain carbohydrates, such as fruits and vegetables, grains, and dairy. Consuming whole foods that contain natural sugar is okay. Plant foods also have high amounts of fiber, essential minerals, and antioxidants, and dairy foods contain protein and calcium.

Since your body digests these foods slowly, the sugar in them offers a steady supply of energy to your cells. A high intake of fruits, vegetables, and whole grains also has been shown to reduce the risk of chronic diseases, such as diabetes, heart disease, and some cancers.

However, problems occur when you consume too much added sugar—that is, sugar that food manufacturers add to products to increase flavor or extend shelf life.

In a study published in 2014 in *JAMA Internal Medicine*, Dr. Hu and his colleagues found an association between a high-sugar diet and a greater risk of dying from heart disease. Over the course of the fifteen-year study, people who got 17–21 percent of their calories from added sugar had a 38 percent higher risk of dying from cardiovascular disease compared with those who consumed 8 percent of their calories as added sugar.

In the American diet, the top sugar sources are soft drinks, fruit drinks, flavored yogurts, cereals, cookies, cakes, candy, and most processed foods. But added sugar is also present in items that you may not think of as sweetened, like soups, bread, cured meats, and ketchup.

There are at least 61 different names for sugar.

From sucrose, which is table sugar, to high-fructose corn syrup, which is liquid sugar, food producers have come up with a plethora of ways to list this nutrient on labels. This makes it even easier to skim over a long ingredient name in a shopping hurry and inadvertently take in more sugar than you meant to (https://www.womenshealthmag.com/food/a19981764/different-names-for-sugar/).

Lustig says that food manufacturers often list different types of added sugars as the seventh, eighth, and ninth items on an ingredient list to fool you into thinking there's not a significant number of added sweeteners. "When you add it up, it's number 1," he says. Pretty sneaky—and scary.

"Sugar can act like poison in high doses—and the amount in our diets has gone beyond toxic," says Robert Lustig, MD, a neuroendocrinologist at the University of California at San Francisco School of Medicine. The typical American now swallows the equivalent of twenty-two sugar cubes every twenty-four hours. When eaten in such vast quantities, sugar can wreak havoc on the body. Over time, that havoc can lead to diabetes and obesity, and also Alzheimer's disease and breast, endometrial, and colon cancers. One new study found that normal-weight people who loaded up on sugar doubled their risk of dying from heart disease.

"No doubt about it," says Hyman. "We're sweetening ourselves sick, yet screaming for more. Why? Because we're seriously hooked. Research shows that hyper-sweet foods may be as addictive as the hardest-to-quit drugs."

Watch for these sneaky ingredients when reading food labels. Some sound scientific, some almost healthy—but in the end, they all mean "sugar."

- Agave nectar
- Barbados sugar
- Barley malt syrup
- Beet sugar
- Blackstrap molasses
- Cane crystals
- Cane juice crystals
- Castor sugar
- Corn sweetener
- Corn syrup
- Corn syrup solids
- Crystalline fructose
- Date sugar
- Demerara sugar
- Dextrose
- Evaporated cane juice
- Florida crystals
- Fructose
- Fruit juice
- Fruit juice concentrate
- Galactose
- Glucose
- Glucose solids
- Golden sugar
- Golden syrup
- Granulated sugar
- Grape juice concentrate
- Grape sugar
- High-fructose corn syrup
- Honey
- Icing sugar
- Invert sugar

- Lactose
- Malt syrup
- Maltodextrin
- Maltose
- Mannitol
- Maple syrup
- Molasses
- Muscovado syrup
- Organic raw sugar
- Powdered sugar
- Raw sugar
- Refiners' syrup
- Rice syrup
- Sorbitol
- Sorghum syrup
- Sucrose
- Table sugar
- Treacle
- Turbinado sugar
- Yellow sugar

If you have a sweet tooth like I do, then I have sweet news! Unless it's all you eat, it's hard to go overboard with truly natural sugars that come directly from fruits and some veggies. Here's the trick: You have to eat the produce. Fruit juices, even those without added sweeteners, will still sugar-bomb your bloodstream. The key is in the fiber, which slows sugar's absorption in your body, preventing an insulin spike. Any fruit is fair game. "Ones with the most natural sugar also have the most fiber," says Robert Lustig, MD.

The percentage of cocoa solids can affect the magnitude of dark chocolate's benefits. "The higher percentage of cocoa solids, the more flavonoids and the lower sugar. If you're doing 75 percent or 80 percent dark chocolate, there'll be less added sugar than if you were at 50 percent dark chocolate."

I gave up M&M's, Snickers, and everything else that melts, and now eat oranges after I wash the toxins off. I find it easy to eat about three per day. I also enjoy 85 to 100 percent dark chocolate since it has so many important minerals, is high in fiber, antioxidants, and flavonoids, which relax blood vessels and improve blood flow. I don't eat a lot of dark chocolate, but I like to treat myself now and then and eat a handful of almonds and Brazil nuts to go along with it.

CHAPTER 11

Foods in the Bible

You are now entering the nice chapters in the book. After all, as I told my grandchildren, if God made the food, then it's good for you. So after reading in the previous chapters about how humans altered God's food by using chemicals, GMOs, or hormones, you're now going to see the better choice, especially since everything God created is good.

Apple: This nutritious fruit offers multiple health benefits. Apples may lower your chance of developing cancer, diabetes, and heart disease. Research says apples may also help you lose weight while improving your gut and brain health.

Figs offer benefits but might also cause other ailments. Best to talk to a nutritionist or doctor before taking figs.

Olives are a staple of the Mediterranean diet. They're associated with many health benefits, especially for heart health and cancer prevention.

Fish: "Of all the creatures living in the water, you may eat any that has fins and scales" (Deuteronomy 14:9). My favorite is wild-caught salmon, which has so many nutritional benefits.

Bread: When bread is mentioned in the Bible, it is at a time when foods were not processed or included additives. Instead, it was made from all-natural ingredients.

The meats did not have hormones or GMOs. They grazed and ate natural foods.

- Goat
- Oxen
- Lamb
- Sheep
- Venison

CHAPTER 12

My Cup of Tea

- Ginger
- Turmeric
- Cinnamon
- Honey—Although not a spice, I found honey had cancer-fighting capabilities, so I decided to make my own tea using these ingredients. I love the taste and usually drink two mugs per day. The listed spices I found to also fight off cancer, colds, and the flu as well as supporting my immune system.

THERE ARE SO many spices out there that are so good for you. If you want the family to learn about the benefits of spices, tell them to bring all the spices you have. Let each person be assigned a certain spice until all the spices are assigned. Then each person will research the benefits the spice offers. My grandchildren were amazed to learn my tea is helping me fight cancer as well as colds and the flu. They then wanted to know about the other spices I had and what they could do. If you have a disease that you're concerned with, your research can be what spices fight against whatever disease you're concerned with.

I believe modern medicine is wonderful and needed, but I also believe we can play an important role in our health with what we eat. My hope is that it may help us in our fight against disease or at least slow it down by eating the right foods and strengthening our immune system.

Again, I'm not an expert, but I do have hope. I believe God provides us with so many good natural foods, herbs, and spices that can boost our immune system and fight disease. I also learned that some spicy foods could slow the growth of cancer.

CHAPTER 13

Herbs and Spices

I COULDN'T WAIT to get to this chapter since the health benefits of herbs and spices are rarely discussed or encouraged, so I was anxious to learn. I will say up front that some herbs and spices may cause problems with certain medications; in fact, various herbs and spices may have better results than some medications. So, I suggest visiting a naturopath, nutritionist, or your doctor who can provide better guidance than I can. I just want to inform you of perhaps an alternative and healthier choice. Various studies have shown that some spices and herbs used as seasoning can strengthen your immune system. I believe a strong immune system is our best first line of defense to fight disease. After all, diseases start small, and at their weakest point is when our immune system should kill the disease. I also believe having a weak immune system allows diseases, at their weakest point, to strengthen. I don't know if studies can prove that, but it just makes too much sense to me, and I didn't want to ignore it.

To start my research, I decided to look in our own pantry to see what spices and herbs we have and learn the health benefits of each. I was amazed at what I found. Garlic, ginger, cinnamon, basil, cloves, parsley, turmeric, oregano, and cilantro all have wonderful health benefits. But since allergies and medications may have negative effects on your body, I suggest contacting a professional to be certain they're safe for you. I believe you'll be surprised by the health benefits of the spices and herbs in your own pantry. This can be a fun family project that even grandchildren might be proud to be involved in. Maybe their involvement will encourage them to eat healthier by adding their favorite spice to a meal, or perhaps they can make their own special tea.

My research has given me new hope while battling this deadly glioblastoma, stage 4, brain cancer. When people are dealing with an incurable, terminal cancer, finding new hope generates a wonderful feeling, unlike the feeling I had when seeing the healthy foods I was eating listed on the Dirty Dozen with the most toxins. That feeling was so discouraging. But I now have new hope again, because now I know better, and I stay away from toxic food. Anyway, I thought I should share my experience since cancer patients are all in this together, and together, we fight! We must have hope and believe what we're doing is beneficial. I believe what I'm doing is helping me, and having that belief is comforting.

My wife is not only a wonderful person but an awesome cook too, who uses herbs and spices often. It allows me to believe I'm putting great nutrients in my body to help fight disease and strengthen my immune system. Besides, the food tastes great.

Since so many herbs and spices exist, I didn't list them all; however, information is just a click away if you want to do your research. A personal example of my research is trying to find what herb or spice can improve eye health and brain function and fight cancer. So many health benefits out there that I never knew existed. I pray you find new hope.

I used some URLs to provide additional information. I hope you enjoy the benefits as much as I do. (https://www.hopkinsmedicine.org/health/wellness-and-prevention/5-spices-with-healthy-benefits).

Turmeric

One of the components of turmeric is a substance called curcumin. Research suggests it may reduce inflammation in the brain, which has been linked to Alzheimer's disease and depression. In a small study of adults over 50, those who consumed curcumin supplements over the course of 18 months had improvement in memory test scores. They also reported being in better spirits. Most impressive? Scans of their brain indicated significantly fewer markers associated with cognitive decline.

Because of its anti-inflammatory qualities, curcumin is also effective at reducing pain and swelling in people with arthritis. And animal studies indicate that curcumin could have powerful anti-cancer properties. A Johns Hopkins study found that a combination of curcumin and a chemotherapy drug was more effective at shrinking drug-resistant tumors than using chemotherapy alone.

Coriander (https://www.webmd.com/diet/health-benefits-coriander).

The vitamins, minerals, and antioxidants in coriander provide significant health benefits. Coriander leaves and seeds are full of vitamin K, which plays an important role in helping your blood clot.

Vitamin K also helps your bones repair themselves, helping prevent problems like osteoporosis. Additionally, evidence points to vitamin K helping lower your risk of heart disease.

Coriander is full of antioxidants, which are important for fighting free radicals in your body. Free radicals are loose oxygen molecules that can damage your cells, potentially causing cancer, heart disease, and more.

Please see your doctor or nutritionist before taking since they may have a negative effect on pregnancy or certain medications. Doing your own research will be rewarding too. The following herbs and spices fight cancer, strengthen the immune system and are good for heart health:

- Rosemary
- Basil
- Sage
- Oregano
- Cilantro
- Parsley
- Dill
- Thyme

- Fennel
- Tarragon
- Garlic
- Ginger
- Chives
- Cayenne Pepper
- Turmeric
- Peppermint
- Marjoram
- Lemon Balm
- Cumin
- Bay Leaf
- Fenugreek
- Lavender
- Mint
- Cinnamon
- Olive Leaf
- Oregano
- Black Pepper
- Saffron
- Coriander

Ginger

Research has found that ginger is effective at calming pregnancy-related nausea and reducing tummy upset after surgery. Some studies have also found that ginger cuts the severity of motion sickness or prevents the symptoms altogether. It may even help with chemotherapy-induced nausea and vomiting when taken along with anti-nausea medications. (Ask your doctor first before taking ginger while on chemotherapy drugs, as it can have a negative interaction with certain medications.)

Garlic

Most of us are familiar with garlic, the strong-smelling bulb frequently used in cooking. But what you might not know is that eating garlic may protect your heart from changes that lead to heart disease.

As you age, some hardening of the arteries is normal. This is called atherosclerosis and occurs as fatty deposits made up of cholesterol and other substances build up on the inside of your artery walls. Factors such as smoking, high blood pressure, and high cholesterol can make it worse. As the buildup increases over time, the arteries narrow. This can make you susceptible to heart attacks and strokes.

Researchers have linked garlic intake with keeping blood vessels flexible, especially in women. In addition, studies suggest that eating garlic may reduce cholesterol and triglycerides.

Peppermint (https://www.medicalnewstoday.com/articles/healthy-herbs-and-spices#peppermint).

An extremely popular herb that is commonly used as a flavoring agent, peppermint is native to Europe and Asia. In these regions, people used it before the advent of modern medicine for its cooling effects, antibacterial properties and to improve digestive health.

Research shows that as a holistic remedy, peppermint is also effective in improving cardiovascular (heart) and pulmonary (lung) health by acting as a bronchodilator. Bronchodilators work by widening air passages (bronchioles) in the lungs. By inhaling the smell of peppermint, a person will also increase their nasal air force, in turn supplying more air to the lungs.

Cinnamon

Ancient civilizations have used cinnamon since 2,800 BCE for anointing, embalming, and treating ailments. Though not as widely used for its therapeutic properties as it was thousands of years ago, cinnamon still provides a myriad of health benefits as an antimicrobial, antioxidant, anti-inflammatory, antidiabetic, and anticarcinogenic spice. Cinnamon may also provide heart-healthy benefits, such as reducing high blood cholesterol and triglyceride levels. That's especially important for people with diabetes who are at greater risk for developing heart disease.

Cinnamon is not a replacement for diabetes medication or a carbohydrate-controlled diet, but it can be a helpful addition to a healthy lifestyle.

Chili Powder

When it comes to cardiovascular benefits, recent research provided by the American Heart Association found that those who regularly consume chili powder may reduce their risk of developing heart disease mortality by 26 percent. Additionally, frequent chili consumption correlates with a 25 percent reduction in mortality from any cause and 23 percent fewer cancer deaths.

Thanks to its anti-inflammatory properties, chili powder could also be effective for supporting arthritis treatments, as well as for alleviating muscle and joint inflammation.

Parsley

Parsley offers many health benefits and contains cancer-fighting substances. In addition, it supports the immune system and bone and eye health, improves heart health, and is rich in antioxidants. It can also reduce blood pressure.

Peppercorn

Piperine, a naturally occurring compound that gives peppercorns their kick, may reduce the risk of certain cancers, including those of the breast, lung, prostate, ovaries, and digestive tract, according to a 2019 *Applied Sciences* review. There are several mechanisms at play, but one of the key benefits of piperine is that it can trigger apoptosis, a biochemical process that tells cells to self-destruct before they have the chance to grow out of control and form tumors.

Cloves

Cloves are also a great source of beta-carotene, which is what gives them their rich, dark brown color. In the body, beta-carotene is converted into vitamin A—an important nutrient for keeping our eyes healthy.

Oregano

Oregano is rich in antioxidants, which are compounds that help fight damage from harmful free radicals in the body.
The buildup of free radicals has been linked to chronic diseases like cancer and heart disease.

Chives

Vegetables are excellent sources of healthy nutrients. Chives contain a range of beneficial nutrients that may offer some health benefits, including anticancer effects.
This chapter made me feel more confident because I believe it provides additional hope to not only fight stage 4 terminal brain cancer but many other diseases too. I love the tea that I make; it tastes great, fights cancer, and builds my immune system. But I think I'm going to add some mint to it, because that, too, is beneficial in my battle to fight cancer. Besides, maybe it'll taste better since I like mint.

CHAPTER 14

Omega-3 Fatty Acids

(https://my.clevelandclinic.org/health/
articles/17290-omega-3-fatty-acids)

What do omega-3 fatty acids do?

OMEGA-3 FATTY ACIDS help all the cells in your body function as they should. They're a vital part of your cell membranes, helping to provide structure and supporting interactions between cells. While they're important to all your cells, omega-3s are concentrated in high levels in cells in your eyes and brain.

What are the benefits of omega-3 fatty acids?

Omega-3 fatty acids have many potential benefits for your cardiovascular health. One key benefit is that they help lower your triglyceride levels. Too many triglycerides in your blood (hypertriglyceridemia) raise your risk of atherosclerosis and, through this, can increase your risk of heart disease and stroke. So it's important to keep triglyceride levels under control.

In addition, omega-3s may help you by raising your HDL (good) cholesterol and lowering your blood pressure. Omega-3 fatty acids may lower your cardiovascular disease risk when you consume them as part of your diet. In general, it's better to opt for food sources (like fish) rather than pills (https://health.clevelandclinic.org/the-best-sources-of-omega-3-fatty-acids).

Omega-3 Fatty Acid Fish

- Herring: 1.7 grams per 3 ounces
- Wild salmon: 1.6 grams per 3 ounces
- Bluefin tuna: 1.3 grams per 3 ounces
- Mackerel: 1 gram per 3 ounces
- Sardines: 0.9 grams per 3.75-ounce can
- Anchovies: 0.9 grams per 2-ounce can
- Lake trout: 0.8 grams per 3 ounces
- Striped bass: 0.8 grams per 3 ounces

If you're wondering about canned tuna, try to limit the amount you eat, as it can contain high levels of mercury. Stick to the chunky light option for reduced mercury amounts. That's especially important if you're pregnant or nursing, which means you should avoid other high-mercury fish too, like swordfish, shark, and tilefish.

It's always best to consult your doctor before major changes to your diet, even healthy ones. This way, you can avoid any complications from allergies. Plus, your doctor knows what approaches and foods will work best for you and your specific health situation.

CHAPTER 15

Beef: Grass-Fed versus Grain-Fed

GRASS-FED BEEF, AS the name implies, comes from cows that eat mostly grass.

Grain-fed cows eat a diet that includes soy, corn, and other additives. Grain-fed cows may also be given antibiotics and growth hormones to fatten them up quickly. I try to stay away from this type of meat source because of the lack of health effects of hormones and additives.

What is Grass-Fed Meat, Omega-3?

(https://medicalhealthauthority.com/info/benefits-of-grass-fed-omega-3.html)

Grass-fed omega-3 refers to the omega-3 fatty acids found in the meat and dairy products of animals that have been exclusively fed a grass-based diet. These fatty acids are essential for our bodies and play a crucial role in maintaining optimal health.

CHAPTER 16

Fruits and Nuts

PEOPLE OF THE Bible ate many of today's most nutritious "superfoods" in this grouping of fruits and nuts. Pomegranates, for example. Pomegranates are believed to have highly beneficial anti-inflammatory, antioxidant, and anti-tumor properties.

- Apples (Song of Solomon 2:5)
- Almonds (Genesis 43:11; Numbers 17:8)
- Dates (2 Samuel 6:19; 1 Chronicles 16:3)
- Figs (Nehemiah 13:15; Jeremiah 24:1-3)
- Grapes (Leviticus 19:10; Deuteronomy 23:24)
- Melons (Numbers 11:5; Isaiah 1:8)
- Olives (Isaiah 17:6; Micah 6:15)
- Pistachio nuts (Genesis 43:11)
- Pomegranates (Numbers 20:5; Deuteronomy 8:8)
- Raisins (Numbers 6:3; 2 Samuel 6:19)
- Sycamore fruit (Psalm 78:47; Amos 7:14)

CONCLUSION

AFTER SO MUCH research, I believe our most important tool to fight disease and cancer is to have a healthy immune system. However, I found it difficult to build a good immune system when healthy foods have toxins, hormones, or genetically modified organisms (GMOs). After seeing the results of the Dirty Dozen identified by the Environmental Working Group (EWG), I felt the feeling of hope slip away. I lost trust in the FDA, EPA, and USDA for their involvement in why toxic food, hormones, and GMOs are on our dinner tables and why potentially toxic foods are even allowed to be sold at our local stores, especially when the Federal Agencies are not sure of the long-term health effects on humans.

To think outside the box, it seems the FDA funds their own agency. After all, they approve what chemicals can be applied to the foods we eat, what hormones are injected or fed to livestock, and approve plants to be genetically modified. Then to complete the process, they approve the drugs to treat the diseases. I believe the FDA does play an important role in our daily lives, but I just don't see how healthy foods can be labeled healthy anymore when they're listed on the Dirty Dozen list with the most toxins. Perhaps "eat at your own risk" would be a more appropriate label. I could not locate any clinical studies on the effects of consuming pesticide residue on produce or dairy animals with hormones or GMOs in plants.

Since pesticides affect an insect or rodent's nervous system and glioblastoma is a central nervous system cancer, is it a possible or probable cause of why I have glioblastoma, especially since I may have inherited my mother's weak immune system? I don't know, but I believe a study to confirm one way or the other should have been done. The Environmental Working Group was a pleasant surprise.

After all, they provided a list of healthy and uncontaminated foods that allowed me to eat what I now believe are healthy foods. In addition, since herbs and spices have been used medicinally for centuries, I would love to see more information shared and encouraged for use. I also couldn't find any herb or spice clinical studies conducted by the FDA, even though many countries have been using them for centuries.

Additionally, I believe discussions need to occur to determine what will prevent foods with toxins, in or on them, from ever entering our grocery stores and ending up on our dinner tables.

Closing Comments

Although I ran competitively and even built a log cabin, writing and completing this book has become my biggest challenge since I wrote everything while being treated for stage 4 glioblastoma along with poor vision.

Regardless of your faith or belief, I pray you and your family have good health. As for me, I believe in God and His Son, Jesus Christ, who also gives me incredible hope.

If you have a terminal disease, I pray you find your hope and live a long and healthy life.

I do wish you all good health, and hopefully, you found this book informative enough for you and your family to live a healthy life and prevent disease from ever occurring.

May God bless you.

Sincerely,
Alan Fortin

ABOUT THE AUTHOR

ALAN FORTIN HAS been diagnosed with three different types of cancer throughout his lifetime: melanoma, carcinoma, and stage 4 glioblastoma brain cancer. Alan became determined to find possible reasons why he gets various cancers and if he can make improvements to reduce the risk of a fourth cancer. He didn't like reading his last cancer had no cure, only the standard treatment of care. So in spirit, he heard the words, "Write a book." And so the journey began, and he went on a mission to see what he could do. He had to find hope, especially since the medical field doesn't offer much for glioblastoma patients. He believes he found it, but that, too, involves risk, but only if you're not aware.